ONE-BREASTED WOMAN

ONE-BREASTED WOMAN

POEMS BY
SUSAN DEBORAH KING

HOLY COW! PRESS • DULUTH, MINNESOTA • 2007

Thanks to the editors of *Minnesota Monthly*, in which the poem
"Foods of a Lifetime" first appeared.

Library of Congress Cataloging-in-Publication Data

King, Susan Deborah.
One-breasted woman : poems / by Susan Deborah King.
p. cm.
ISBN 978-0-9779458-2-5 (alk. paper)
1. Breast — Cancer — Poetry.   1. Title.
PS3611.I586O53 2007
811'.6—DC22   2007004485

This project was supported by a major grant from the
George Family Foundation, with additional contributions provided by
the Alan H. Zeppa Family Foundation, the Reheal Fund —
Roger Hale/Nor Hall of The Minneapolis Foundation,
and by individual donors.

Holy Cow! Press books are distributed to the trade by
Consortium Book Sales & Distribution, c/o Perseus Distribution,
1094 Flex Drive, Jackson, Tennessee 38301.

For personal inquiries, write to:
Holy Cow! Press,
Post Office Box 3170
Mount Royal Station
Duluth, Minnesota 55803
Please visit our website: www.holycowpress.org

for Penny George,

Polly Bunker

and, of blessed memory,

Esther Rome

TABLE OF CONTENTS

PREFACE

AFTER A DIAGNOSIS of breast cancer in 1999 at age 51 and undergoing a mastectomy of my right breast as treatment for this disease, I found that, as a poet, writing about what I was experiencing came naturally as a way to quell the rising tide of terror that rose up in me. It was a way too to feel that I was *doing* something in relation to my illness (the Greek root of the word "poetry" is the verb meaning *to do* or *to make*). Just the *making* itself reduced my anxiety and provided a kind of solace. Since poetry, the most concentrated form of language, in the earliest human times, probably took the form of spells to ensure the success of a hunt and hence the survival of the tribe, I sensed at a very primal level that engaging in spell-making might have a positive effect on my state of being, even my survival. I needed to catch the torrent of feeling unleashed by the experience in many vessels, vessels made of words, so it would not overcome me, so it might be *contained* and have a chance, under the heat of attention and meditation, to turn into a healing balm. The raw emotion that surfaces in an encounter with the possibility of imminent death, the disfigurement and vulnerability inherent in the breast cancer experience called forth from me a kind of strength and capacity for living more fully in whatever time I'm given and forged for me a deeper and broader connection with other humans and all forms of life. The process of diagnosis, treatment and recovery and the writing about it was indeed a transformative one, leaving me with an abiding sense of poignancy about our life's brevity, gratitude for it and even joy.

To describe and frame this experience of transformation, I have chosen terms, which I consider particularly apt, from the discipline of alchemy to announce the three sections of this book. C. G. Jung, the psychologist, and his followers studied the ancient art/science of alchemy and found that it described very well what many undergo numerous times in the course of psychoanalysis and individuation: a movement from despair/ illness/dissolution to awakening/ purification/ emergence to fulfillment/joy/actualization. These three stages: *nigredo, albedo, rubedo*, correspond to the colors black, white and red. In alchemy, the adept takes the dark, confusing, horrifying material of suffering and pours it into a vessel, raises the heat under it till it cooks and changes color, changes quality from the white of rising consciousness to the red of full realization.

Let's say that the adept in this book is One-Breasted Woman. She is a figure larger than myself who visited me in the course of this ordeal. She is possessed of a powerful and passionate vulnerability. She raises up with outrage the possible systemic causes of her disease ("Biological Survey Map, Stearns County, Minnesota"), and she holds the earth ("Elm") and beloved people close ("Being Read *Wind in the Willows*") as she contemplates her end ("As Death Approaches...") and connects with the suffering of others ("Epidemic"). She presides over the frightening material bubbling in the vessel until it changes and redeems itself ("Crucible"). As Marie-Louise von Franz, a colleague of Jung's, has said, "Sitting in Hell and roasting there brings forth the philosopher's stone." That stone is the goal of the alchemical process. ("Agate Hunting") Despite whatever conflicts rage or trouble assails, if one has chosen consciously to endure, to pay attention to suffering and not try to escape it. something solid, immoveable and quiet can form and hold at the center of oneself.

Before I was diagnosed with breast cancer, I had no idea how prevalent is this disease. Every 1.9 minutes a woman is diagnosed with breast cancer, and every 13 minutes someone dies from it. There can be hardly a soul who has not known someone affected in some way by this affliction, let alone all the other cancers that occur. And yet, as soon as one is told one actually has cancer, a kind of loneliness descends that is like no other. The world divides into those who have cancer and those who don't; those who are facing the prospect of imminent death, and those who can still maintain the illusion they don't have to right now. Into my loneliness came an angel: Penny George, someone I had met through my husband's work earlier the same year as my diagnosis. I knew she had struggled with 3rd stage invasive breast cancer and had recovered through chemotherapy and the practice of many non-traditional alternative therapies. As a result of her experience, she had decided to leave her practice in industrial psychology in order to head her family's foundation, making its mission that of promoting the practice of integrative medicine; that is, using and validating alternative healing methods such as meditation, yoga, acupuncture, ritual, vision quest and practice in the arts alongside traditional Western medical models.

Penny visited me during my short hospital stay and unselfconsciously showed me her prosthesis. She gave me information about how to obtain one for myself and suggested I participate in a group at Virginia Piper Medical Center that was led by a healing coach funded by her foundation. More than that, Penny became someone in whom I could confide my worst fears. It is hard for one's family to hear all one feels at such a time. She was very present company in my darkness. As I continued to process my experience and the poems began to come, I shared them with her.

One day in early 2002, I received a call from her foundation office asking if a grant from them would help me complete this set of poems. Penny knew that my teaching schedule made it hard for me to devote the time I'd like to the poems. Thanks to her and the George Family Foundation, I was able to cut back on teaching for awhile so I could complete this manuscript. Most of these poems developed within the three years following my illness, though some kept coming over time as I began to come to grips with how having breast cancer had altered my life and my priorities and had shifted my spiritual perspective. I will be forever grateful to her and the Foundation for this opportunity. It is my hope that this book might provide some measure of the company she offered to me during my dark journey through cancer, so that those who read this will feel less lonely as they travel.

I experienced companionship in the depths as well from the work of other writers and artists, who had been diagnosed with breast cancer or had faced other life-threatening illnesses or situations: Lucille Clifton, Naomi Shihab Nye, Thich Nhat Hanh, Tulku Thondup, Charlotte Joko Beck, Esther Rome and the Boston Women's Health Book Collective, Kat Duff, Lu Ann Lewis and her sculpted mastectomy angels, Hilda Raz's anthology *Living on the Margins*, Judith Lief's *Making Friends with Death*, an anthology of art and writing about breast cancer: *Art. Rage. Us.*, Audre Lorde's *The Cancer Journals*, and especially Rachel Naomi Remen's *Kitchen Table Wisdom*.

Other sister survivors I would like to thank for the comfort of their company are Polly Bunker, Chris Morrow and her art, Jo Calhoun, Renee Macomber, Martie Van Roekel, Roseanne Monten, Dorothy Silvers, Emily Nelligan, Peggy Sanford, and Hallee Wannamaker. I am very grateful to Diane Neimann, head of staff at the George Foundation and to Lora Matz, the healing coach at that time at Virginia Piper, who led a healing group using ritual, art, music and craft. I resisted entering this group because I was angry and afraid. She urged me to join, and thank heaven I finally accepted the invitation. (Note: Those who are part of groups of people struggling with cancer have a 40% greater chance of survival and recovery than those who don't.) Thanks to Ann Chapman who led me to Franklin Dennis, who helped this book find a home and to Jim Perlman at Holy Cow! Press, who took it on. Thanks very much to Polly Brody for her friendship and for going over this manuscript with her excellent fine-toothed comb, to Jolinda Osborne, who offered friendship too and special help, to Ralph Henn and to Susan Thornton, who was my pastor through my illness and beyond. Thanks too to four physicians whose uncommon kindliness of manner went well beyond standard medical practice to contribute to my healing: Drs. Carolyn Cody, Charles Hendricks, Ruth Dietz and Richard Zera. Thanks especially to many, many friends who sustained me with their presence and their prayers and for my family: Jim, Emily and Enid, who saw me through. At this writing, I am cancer-free, healthy, and very glad to be alive.

Susan Deborah King
Minneapolis, January, 2007

(She) deposes doom
who hath suffered Him
    Emily Dickinson

WHERE SHE CAN BE FOUND

Off the track, by the sea,
in a camp with breathing walls,
hanging out with her snake
and her dog. They find her safe.
There's always a fire going,
a cup of brew for passers through:
the whole crew: bruised, cuckoo,
ruined, lonely, exhausted.
She literally lives on love,
all the nurture she needs.

She doesn't care a stick anymore
how she, or anyone else, looks.
What would be the point?
Down to her spreading hips falls
her wild, wavy gray mane,
yet she can be glimpsed at night
through candlelit panes trying on
ribbons and capes, enjoying jewels.

When she needs a good laugh –
and who doesn't in this brutal world? –
she looks in the glass. What she sees
is a lovely, lumpy, lopsided hag.
And what a laugh: burble, warble,
cackle, gasp – rat-a-tat-tat, sometimes
hard to distinguish from weeping – or fury.

Mornings on the porch she sits and mulls,
tunes her ears to the birds and tides,
watches light play and change among the trees,
wind lifting, then settling the leaves.
She rolls a stone in her hand.
She praises her blooms.
Every day she makes a little something
to offer in thanks, a long skinny lime green
prayer flag for a soul in grief, a bright,
multicolored mat to go under daily plates.

At some point she jumps up, charges out,
hobbles down halls of power at a clip
to hector legislators for the air, fair treatment,
healing, housing, for schools, for food,
against attacks – all
for the sake of the *child*.
What we would care more about,
she can't fathom.

NIGREDO

Only out of utmost darkness and loss and despair do we come to ourselves.
        Elizabeth Boyden Howes, *The Choicemaker*

Insecurity we need perhaps the most when we are inventing.
        Mary Caroline Richards, *In Pottery, Poetry and Person*

The greatest kind of courage. The courage to be afraid.
        Helene Cixous, *Coming to Writing and Other Essays*

SONG SPARROW

Showing how it's done,
he perches right before me
on a bare spruce branch,
bold as brass. Though his breast
has a black mark on it,
he throws his head back
and with quivering throat,
open beak, sends out
his clear, trill-finished phrase.
He is not deterred because
he lacks a warbler's yellow dash,
its more sophisticated tune,
nor because his life is short
and no one will remember him
when he goes. It is Spring.
It is just past dawn.
I am here! he exclaims.
This melody: sweet, sweet, sweet,
these streaks, this tweedy cape.
This is who I am.
I am.

FLOWERS

for Ashley Bryan

They thrust buds into rain
allowing sun
to unseal their sepals.
They peel back
expose their colors,
their tender, tentacled centers
for bees to ransack, plundering
bags bulging with gold.
Plucky, profligate,
they extend themselves,
offer the wind their leaves,
their petals, not chagrinned
to flutter, to tremble,
not picky, not wishing
a different season, a better,
they hold nothing back,
as if *this* is it,
NOW!

Busting open with panache,
full blast, they seem almost
to launch, to lunge toward
their deaths
even as, shriveling,
they cast abroad their seeds,
bequeathing them, whether
it receives them or not,

to the earth. Some,
like comets streaking the heavens,
carry ahead their forms,
plant their pennons,
splendiferous,
beyond.

CRUCIBLE

When heated directly by fire,
the fire of trial, the heat of disease,
infernos of grief and penury,
the clay we're made of,
will it crack and shatter,
or thicken against the blaze
a shield – refractory, infusible?
Will our flesh create a vessel
for all that is cold and hard,
marred, opposed, outmoded
to melt – the hotter the flame,
forms sloughed, the more
molten we'll become,
the more in flux, the more
to the crux? Can we
hold under the terror,
the torment of transforming,
under forging
until we are
bearers of light, torches,
for sufferance,
for illumining
oblivion?

TULIPS DYING

The household into which they were brought
as a gift – pink, lavender splashes
against February grime – is much too
overwrought to pay them mind. Lately,
the occupants have speeded up: answering email,
real mail, calls off the machine, recycling,
faxing, xeroxing, nuking Lean Cuisine,
pouring coffee into travel mugs, before,
way behind, dashing off. No chance
for glances at blowzy heads craning
at this rush, the disarray in its wake,
their supple, slightly bended stems
sucking up darkening water in the vase,
soft green leaf spears arcing over the lip.
Their petals' silken flesh dries and twists
to parchment, to husks. Now they could be
arthritic fingers straining for one last grasp,
or bodies frozen in macabre arabesques.
It will be days before anyone notices
and in disgust absentmindedly tosses them
into dark plastic bags with moldy applesauce
to await the garbage truck's uproarious jaws.

BLACK PELICANS

for Polly Brody

Sharper-eyed than I,
from a bluff over the great river
that splits this continent in half,
you spot them way down.
Closer in your high-powered
glasses, a squadron heading toward us,
but so far off, they all look black,
together, undulating –
a waving handkerchief.
Good-bye or hello?
Surely, they'll never reach us.
They'll veer off, switch direction,
double back. I'm waiting
for the results of tests,
an X-rayed mass.
As always, you stand by me
on the look out.
It appears they're following
the river's course,
straight up.
How much time do we have?
Minutes, you judge.
Couldn't we just stop,
and hold here, in this gift
companionship, anticipant,
with Spring all around us
unclenching yellow-green fists?

My God! Suddenly,
they're huge!
Wings nine feet across
like trireme oars
rowing the blue.
Bombers with a payload.
I see now their bodies are white,
only their primaries
black and up-tipped
like Japanese gateway lintels.
They approach as one,
a kinetic cloud,
level with the bluff
so near they could easily
scoop us into their
big yellow pouches.
What seemed so far off,
what would never,
has come upon us:
the Most High,
as they pass,
overshadowing.

CANCER

Cancer cells are out of control.
They're abnormal, deranged.
They divide excessively.
They're obsessed with growth.
They divide excessively.
That's abnormal. That's deranged!
They keep rhyming themselves:
Their numbers swell.
No one knows how.
Cancer cells are out of control.
Their numbers swell.
They invade other tissues.
Take over whole organs,
and shut them down.
They're out of control,
deranged, abnormal.
They're obsessed with growth.
Take over whole countries.
They drive up the Dow, the GNP.
Cancer cells are out of control.
Rhyming themselves,
dividing excessively.
Consuming all nutrients,
all sources of energy.
Rhyming, griming, sliming – thriving!
Heeding no warnings.
Ice caps melting, the loss of the wild.

A chunk, the size of Texas,
calving from the ice shelf.
Cancer cells ignore controls.
They're obsessed with growth.
The last "first contact" was years ago.
Car hulks pile up.
Out of control.
Deranged, abnormal!
Consuming, consuming.
70 species extinct each day.
70 species extinct each day.
They invade all terrains.
Consuming all nutrients,
they progress. They make progress.
"Immortal," unstoppable,
their numbers swell.
No one knows how,
though we study and study,
they take over and kill,
ignoring all warnings,
take over and kill
the whole body,
the whole globe,
the whole body.
Out of control!

BIOLOGICAL SURVEY MAP, STEARNS COUNTY, MN

What would the world be, once bereft, of wet and wildness?
from "Inversnaid" by Gerard Manley Hopkins

Belt buckle of the state we can't help
thinking is shaped like a lopsided human torso,
this county, large and largely rural, what we think of
as "the country," only 1.6% of its area is
covered by native plantings now. Color coded:
green for upland and riverbottom forests;
brown for oak openings, barrens; orange
for brush lands; pink for marshes, meadows, fens;
swamps and bogs in purple, a map that
in 1857 was every inch a festal mix of colors,
today is almost entirely white.

Only 150 years it took us to cut this land
like sheet cake into township squares
and gobble it down, dropping scanty crumbs.
There are just too many of us.
We swarm like the grasshoppers
that ravaged my childhood farm
leaving only peach pits dangling from branches.
Hereabouts, a story goes, a scourge like that
was averted by very pious German Catholic prayers.

Unequipped with such, clutches of trees
huddle together at the edge of a field,
ripped up sod become an ever-furrowed brow.

Nowhere enough of them to qualify any more
as woods. You can see right through them
to the next wave of crops, to treeless plots
with vinyl-sided ranches, satellite dishes,
swing sets with loud plastic slides,
synthetic blue above-ground pools.

Gaping quarry holes, granite gouged out
for floors, coasters, countertops; long,
scarcely-vented turkey coops, doghouse-sized
cramps for veal calves; garages, mammoth, of
corrugated metal for hoes and dozers
that tear roads through turf and roots; towers
of exes, red beams bleeping on top.
Doesn't our species deserve to eat and prosper?

A thick, serpentine stand of tamaracks is
the only significant holdout here against us
its feet planted in muck, too forbidding
to develop. Shoulder to shoulder, they present
their delicate bristles until, in autumn,
they drop, a staunch, outnumbered red-gold
battalion, a natural world Massadah or Musa Dagh.

for Hal Watson

RED

Red scares me.
Shouldn't it?
The color of stop.
Stop signs, stop lights,
emergency, danger.
Too much red –
it hurts my eyes.
It gets inside me.
I went to her house
after she died.
Everything was red:
the sheets, the towels,
the walls, the drapes,
the rugs, the mugs,
knife handles, lamp shades,
bookends – paperclips!
She had decorated it
after she got sick.
I couldn't sleep in that place.
Even in the dark,
the red closed in
breathed hot on my skin.

She wanted to live.
Why couldn't she?
She was mad, real mad,
but she had been taught

to be good
and couldn't show it.
Her love, her blood
was big, too big
for time, for the time
she had. It could have
filled 20 lives,
so the red bled
onto everything
within her reach –
a kind of gory legacy.
She was not ready to go.
No. No!
Red scares me.
Way before we're set,
we can be plucked
right out of our lives.

BEAUTIFUL STORM

It doesn't have to be an oxymoron.
I can see it coming toward us up the coast,
dark, many-mammaried clouds
flashing and growling.
letting down their feeding showers
arced because they're speeding
dense with divesting themselves:
curtains pulling back on theatre earth...
Overhead, a clap, an announcement,
knock-you-down-loud.
The grass heads are nodding, davening,
out of deference, respect,
out of thirst – in thanks.
The red maple is all het up,
then, suddenly, its leaves are slick,
tears, brilliants dripping
from each mahogany tip.
On the pavement, a sauté,
spitting and hissing.
Hot rocks sizzle and cool.
As it recedes, streams of light,
evening light, growth green,
and sky streaks, amongst
ribbons of soot,
blue as the eggs of cormorants.
If only, like so, I could view
my own tumult.

CREDO

All but crazy dreamers
end furiously, grieving hours
in jocularity killed.
Life may not offer purpose,
quirks, ribaldry, susurration,
tolerance unless victim's work
expresses yellow zeal.

BREAST

Sprout stem bud flower
Crest swelling peaks the sea
Billow pillow nipple nuptial
Sun aureole bowl bell
Toll tit tip tongue lips
Sip suck sup spout spile
Sap tapped drink draught
Jug mug vessel cup
Bra clasp hassle erect
Flick kiss pet quick love
Egg sperm germ term
Let down drip dipper tipped
Rooting for milk the moon
Lait de la mer lait de la lune
Thirst for it burst quaff quench
Quest rest fountain mountain
Mosque *mamma* mammary manna
Mother Mom nursing comfort source
Poke probe photo inspect
Source pitted bitten into disease
Face it brave No please! flesh
Slashed scarred forever marred
Whacked off lost gone flung
Waste trash flat concave
Frozen seized grieved aflame

FEMME DE LAVANDE

Of all the *santons*, the people,
the players of a Provençal town,
she is the bringer of purple,
her only purpose to be
the one carrying it in from the field.
She bears it by the armful saying,
Here. Take some sprigs. *Voici!*
Put them between your sheets
so you and your lover can roll
in fragrance, can
cover yourselves as you love
in the perfume of thrumming.
Summer. *L'haut d'ete.*
You have no love, you say?
Find one. Embrace *yourself!*
Depth of shadow. *Couleur de l'ombre.*
Voilà. Take it all.
Take that eventually you will have to
disengage from each other:
He will pull out. You will turn.
You will have to disengage from this world.
La femme wants you to have it,
the falling evening. *Tout. Maintenant!*
Before it fades, before
you wither like the petals.
Sachet is only memory of the flower.
Take it while it's sharp, fresh,

while its cool, harsh *plaisance*
drives a savory shaft down through you,
while its beauty can still wound you
and you bleed *tristesse*.
Now, she dares you,
before you muster
resistance: *Prenez!*

INTERSECTION

How? When? I keep fretting about my death.
Will it stare me down like a threatening stranger?
Will it come from behind, overtake me?
Will it gnaw slowly on my bones or suddenly devour?
What will it feel like? Immersion in warm water? Will I even feel?
And what happens next? Don't such thoughts assault you too?
I've felt so alone, but really we're together.
Aren't we really together, not alone in this?
Don't such thoughts assault you too? About what happens after?
What will it feel like? The ultimate orgasm? Will I even feel?
Will it sink flaming teeth in me or consume me quick like tissue?
Will it come from out of nowhere and sideswipe me?
Will it wear me down with threats, with constant danger?
I can't stop fretting: When? How?

HEAVEN

for JS

The priest sounded so sure,
they'd be waiting there for her,
our friend just gone,
the saints, the martyrs
to give her, because she'd believed
in the One who presides over it,
a gauntlet of welcome.
Embracing and feasting,
merry making, music.
Someday, he said, we might
join her. I think he even thought
he knew the menu.
But would it be that much different
from this party of mourners
gathered now?

Where are we going?
Is the word "where" operative at all,
or words *period*? And,
who am I kidding? *We?*
I feel like our dog shaking
in the car all the way to the vet.
She knows beyond all attempts to soothe:
it's going to hurt.
It's something to fear.
I don't know how to set out
without an idea of a destination,
without the idea of destination.

I don't know how to give up
knowing and wanting to know.

I thought heaven was here
entwined in the naked limbs
of my love, here on this porch
looking out on the sea
among the fragrant, humming grasses,
around the table laughing with friends
eating pilaf and lamb and squash.
I thought it was holding
a homing daughter,
the piercing call
of a white-throated sparrow.
Is earth not heaven enough?
I don't want to leave.

How could there be no me?
What will there be
when I am not?
Will I know
when I go?
Is heaven beyond what we've imagined;
is that its nature, *beyond*,
or do our imaginings
give clues to where we're headed?
Can we trust them at all?
Even now, at best we can just
allow the unfolding.
Each next moment is unknown.
How is stepping into death any different?

EVERYWOMAN'S LEXICON OF DREAD, WITH COMMENTARY (MINIMAL)

Breast Center, routine.
After 50, every year.
At window, *Race for the Cure* registration forms.
Mammogram, mammography, lumps.

Strip to the waist.
Scootch it in. Clamp. Squeeze. *Ouch!*
Hold your breath. Don't breathe!
The machine sounds like a garbage truck grinding junk in its jaws.
Waiting, shivering in a paper bib that makes you sweat,
       that abrades the nipples (still plural).

Suspicious mass. Star against dark ground, brightest spot.
Ultrasound. Warm gel slathered on.
Anything white: mass, tumor, lesion, growth.
Radiologist reading the film – nurse,
Don't worry they often overread. –
Maybe just a calcification.

Biopsy scheduled. Needle biop. Stereotactic.
Lying face down. Slot in a donut
where the breast drops through.
Hangs vulnerable. Like teats in a milking parlor.
Lidocane not enough.
Deep in tissue. Jab. Jerk!
A lot of blood. Over the PA,

too loud, Andrea Bocelli, "Time to Say Good-bye"
After a two week wait, *We don't mean to alarm you.*
Papilloma. 10-20% chance malignant.
Ectomies. Omas.

Lumpectomy. Wire Loc. *What is **that**?*
It's just like a fish hook.
Deep in the breast. Protrudes 6".
Dixie cup over it while being escorted, gowned, through halls –
  everyone else dressed – to Special Procedures.
Scalpel. Hunk of flesh.
Unpleasant smell? *Don't worry.*
It's just burning flesh.
Your flesh. Like putrid barbequing meat.
Cautery, to stop the bleeding.
Like a piece of lasagna on a marble pallet.
In 48 hours we'll know.

Negative = Positive, Positive = Negative =
Bad.
Clear margins/dirty margins – spread.
*You have ductal carcinoma **in situ**.*
You have cancer.
You have impending death.
We could take the breast or
more lumpectomy, radiation.
Mastectomy, simple mastectomy.
Not radical. Just
the breast itself.
Just
the breast.

Surgery. Hospital. Bracelet,
to identify your corpse.
Anesthesia. *You understand,*
this procedure could lead to your death.
Sign it. Take everything off.
The rings too. Sign them away.
Gown with no secure closures.
Nos morituri te salutamus.
There will be a prick, some stinging.
Propanol. Blankness – total.
Wake from it?

Do wake. To absence, flatness,
one side. Only half. Half a woman.
Incision, drainage, morphine.
Anti-inflammatory. For the burns,
Silvadene cream. (Again cautery)
To a woman in her 30s next to you
behind a curtain, metastasis, inoperable,
you talk, intermittent, into interminable night.
No sleep at all. You feel so close to her — nameless, beautiful
        yet will never see her face.
        Curtain drawn between you.

Drainage bulb fills. Bright red
paling over days. Seroma.
Keeps filling with your fluids.
They don't know anymore where to run.
Pathways blocked.
Then the doc takes the drain out,
a long white plastic serpent,

longer and wider than a multi-plug,
surge-protecting strip.
How in you could there have been room for it?
Scabs. soreness, bunching, scar tissue.
Scar, mouth. Lips sewn shut, bulging.

Beware lymphedema. The arm ballooning.
Climbing up walls
with fingers
restores range of motion.
Let arm hang circling.
Never draw blood from that arm again.
Watch out: Pin pricks, cuts, infection.

Before discharge,
pathology dyes
(pathology = words of suffering, knowledge of pathos)
No residual cancer.
All the above: synonyms for *fear.*
Prognosis: life now.
Death, eventual.

SIMPLE MASTECTOMY, RIGHT BREAST

When I was a teen, it was slow to grow
barely a bump, not ever big enough,
not even big as the other.
I was called flat and filled out only
later, when under stress, I fattened.
Yet, it was the one that ballooned up
twice the size of the left one with
milk, the one from which
I expressed the most
sweet blue fluid to keep the twins
going in neo-natal ICU, the one
that later the littlest sucked,
eagerly, sloppily, droplets
running down from her mouth.
It soaked through nursery pads
to plant a wet circle on my blouse.
How could it harbor anything vile?
It was a twin itself.
I imagine how one of my girls
would feel without the other,
the one left unmatched, part of a
pair lost, unbalanced, forever
calling for the other.
On another level, missing earrings and
socks have always driven me nuts.

It was the one quickest when
licked or flicked to arouse,
the nipple hard, hot wired to
my crotch: secretions
instantly let down, my portal
slickening to abet the making of love.
Now it's gone to a "tissue dump."
Common refuse.
It will never regenerate.
In its place a stitched up slit, lips
pursed to keep from bursting with grief.
Where once a pillow for
husband, friend or child,
now a hollow my daughter nestles into
claiming it's brought us closer.

ASYMMETRY

I am a living sculpture; I am
in-the-flesh performance art.
I resemble classic nudes but for
one noticeable difference.
I have been shaped by the forces of civilization,
a product of progress as any
many-footed frog our rivers cough up.
What for the whole was gain,
for me was abomination.
A piece of me, the softest, sweetest piece,
diseased, lopped off, I become
an inadvertent symbol of your
adoration of perfect surfaces.
To achieve clean lines, some
must let blood, many.
Many are being sacrificed.
I am only one, before you now held up,
as once God, the great symmetry, was.
The sealed and crooked smile,
spreading across the right side of my chest,
challenges your precious balance,
the pinnacle on which it rests.
Outraged, revulsed, you turn your head.
Resist the impulse to center the remaining breast,
to cut it off. Live with the discomfort.
You will learn to find me beautiful
as any Pygmalion who, with his scalpel,

carved the marble
and loved what came to be
of his power, the living proof.

PLASTICS

"It has been determined by a group of eminent doctors and scientists that three things are conclusively carcinogenic. One of them is plastic."
        Maia Sampson

Once we wake naked into the rosy haze of dawn,
where can we turn that they are not?
Our feet land on polyeurethaned hardwood.
As we go about our toilettes, there they are
in almost everything we touch: alarm clock button,
light switch, cup, toothbrush handle, bristles,
lenses, shower curtain, shower cap, razor, bath mat,
synthetic fibered rug; in what we put on:
panties, slip, nylon, rayon – supposedly less
wrinkly than cotton – even our soles are vinyl.

Did you know that softer plastics "gas off,"
release their toxins to whatever comes in contact
with them? It is best not to remember this
as we open the refrigerator, itself fitted out
with plastic components. No element of the breakfast
we fix on a formica counter while standing
on a vinyl-tiled kitchen floor, remains untainted:
Milk jug, plastic-coated juice carton, plastic-lined
cereal box, Saran-wrapped grapefruit half, bread bag,
whole grain or not, garish green margarine tub, melmac.

Why did we abandon ceramics and glass, made from
natural earthen materials? Too heavy, too breakable?
Same with wood and metal, which also rust and de-
compose, and paper that disintegrates when wet.
None but the last are as easy to toss, and
there was, no doubt, money to be made.
Remember the milk bottle? Its graceful shape
and the thick, satisfying cardboard tab at the top.
A washable, reusable icon. Think of the vessels,
the containers other cultures fashioned: Roman
glass, the Greek kalyx, the red-clay Navajo bowl.
Did using them jeopardize people's *health*?

Turning the plastic-headed car key in its lock,
ensconced in polyvinylchloride-covered car seats,
gripping the polyphenylene-oxide wheel,
we grab a quick coffee on the corner, a bottle,
plastic, of pure spring water for later. Setting
the Styrofoam cup in its polystyrene holder,
we try to drive away from thoughts of
how many encounters with plastics we've had
in just this one day's first half hour.

ALBEDO

I wake to sleep and take my waking slow
I learn by going where I have to go.
            Theodore Roethke, "The Waking"

This is the ticket
I failed to spend.
It is still in my pocket
at the fair's end.
It is not only
suffering and grief
or even boredom
of which we are
offered more than
enough.
            Kay Ryan, "Ticket"

ANGELS AND FLOWERS

After the surgery they came flooding
into the house. Vases crowded
every available surface.
To keep them all later, I'd have needed
whole new shelves. *Be well!*
the bursting blossoms shouted;
the colors cried,
We don't want you to leave this earth.
The air was stupendously fragrant.
An unforgettable bouquet of roses
in palest assorted pastels
packed in what seemed an infinite
number of petals, implying
more days, more years.

The angels were mostly handmade:
feathered, papered – holding up
golden banners. One, in clay,
hands on sassy hips
had a mastectomy scar herself.
Another silly one hung over me
shod in outrageous orange boots.
Dearest, from my daughter,
the fuzzy, stuffed, long-billed,
tiny-winged duckling named Murfles.
They kept to my side.
They watched, smiled,

tended the wavering flame of my health.
Did they help?
Love
is the most powerful force in the world.

BEING READ *THE WIND IN THE WILLOWS*

We can't prevent one another from dying.
We can't, though the heart splits apart trying,
will each other to heal. But, read to me –
that you could do, and while the gash
in my chest still oozed, you needed to feel useful.
So I stretched out in the scull of the sofa
and you in the chair beside me, wicker
as Rat's picnic basket, rowed us through
the book we both missed hearing as children,
a chapter each evening as day slipped over
the threshold into the dark. As you spoke
the relish and rollick of its words,
I sank into the boat of the book
and let it carry me down the river of its world,
where animal inhabitants expatiate
on the jolly gifts of water and sky, of snow,
the moon and food by a crackling hearth,
where kindness rules and translates into deeds
and friends, though sometimes dreadfully
peeved, forbear to the end, to redemption,
one another's excesses and believe each
to be good fellows at core.
It was a world not altogether unfamiliar,
so awfully like the one – for I have been
a Toad to your Badger and Rat to your Mole – that,
when lovers are friends, as we have always been,
can actually exist on the earth.

You wanted to ease my passage from it
for both of us, if I should have to go directly,
but in the moments of your reading,
you grew – how could that be? – even dearer.
I was held and clung close,
and the thought, insupportable, of departure,
for that short while at least, dissolved.

BOOB

It's slippery as a bar of wet cartoon soap,
flip-floppy as poorly weighted water toys.
Wearing it, I feel like one.
It looks like a sand dune, a mosque dome,
a homeless mollusk. It shape shifts in my hand
like silly putty, like a piece of meat in aspic.
When prodded, it jiggles. It's a silicone hillock.
When poked, like rising dough, it closes over.
Slipped into this pocketed mastectomy bra,
euphemized, glorified as a Luxa Comfort Form,
Elegant Contours Collection or worse, made
sterile by the technical term "prosthesis,"
it gets warm like a rock in sun. Still warm
for awhile when I take it off as I'll be
for a few moments after I'm gone, it schlumps
faux-nipple down on my bureau making a basin,
a crater, a goblet top – the cup that wouldn't pass.

I could have used a couple of these
at flat-chested thirteen when I picked up this slang
and was told men liked to use them as toys,
but why bother with it now? Because
I don't have the guts to greet the world each day
as an amputee, to have the eyes of people I meet
immediately drift down? Because
I don't want to be identified by loss,
this loathsome fact, as deformed?

Think of the connotations of "unbalanced."
Maybe, against all evidence, I'd like to
maintain the illusion of wholeness.
At least once I'm dressed.

ONE-BREASTED WOMAN

sometimes wishes she could move the one breast
to the center and stretch it so it looks more like two.
Then she would have a strange central nipple,
but she hates being all-to-the-one side and maybe
that would make her feel more balanced.
Maybe it would be like having a third eye.
It might give her special powers of perception
like knowing that being mutilated could open her
to all sorts, all sorts of brokenness she used to ignore.
With it she could sense the integrity of
incompleteness, of impairment, of whoever
is bereft, scathed, wrecked, destitute, mortal.
She could stop trying to find something
somewhere that isn't and might even
learn to celebrate the "as is."

Though, while she's wishing, let's get honest.
She'd just like the other breast back.
She misses cupping them both in her hands,
misses feeling round and ripe and fertile.
She can't bear walking through the bra section.
Bad as going through when she was 12.
Another world that belongs to real women.
Something she'll never need again.
Her bras are those ghastly "bussenhalter" jobs
with the pocket for the falsie she has to get
with a prescription. Young women striding

blithely down the street, their bosoms swaying
gracefully beneath their blouses – she doesn't
begrudge them. She just wants to go up,
look at them hard and ask, *Do you know
what you have?* Can we ever appreciate anything
fully, she wonders, until it's gone for good?

EPIDEMIC

If I thought it would work, I would smear the blood
spilled from me when my breast was removed
over as many lintels and doorposts as I could,
so this plague would pass over those houses.
Again today I picked up my phone
to hear the same heart-tearing news:
suspicious lump and/or conclusive diagnosis.
It's hard not to go numb.
Peggy, Penny, Polly, Jo, Chris, Esther, Ellen.
Betty, Martie, Hallie, Renee, Rhayma, Katherine.
Susie, Mary, Gretchen, Carolyn. Then Colleen
and Nina, mothers of friends of my children.
Now, possibly, even my precious Renita.
Many of these just in the last six months.
And these are only the ones *I* know and love.
Multiply them by everyone who reads this poem.
I want to shout their names into crowds.
Nowhere, as with the plague bubonic,
are the names of the dead, the afflicted,
their numbers published, made widely known.
Daily, even monthly, the facts would run one through.
Perhaps the spread of this is abetted
by rampant silence and denial.
Is that *still* because the victims are "only" women?
I would say it with my blood: No!
A plague – not this, not any – on *none* of your houses.

TWINGES

Once you've had cancer, ever after
every odd sensation is worms
beginning to nibble you.
Jabbing pains, persistent aches
or coughs, cuts slow to heal can be
a witch's finger poking your flesh
to see if you're fat enough yet for the oven,
can be a choking piece of poisoned apple,
a spindle's prick casting an evil spell.

How to trick the witch, get the weight
of her own ego to throw her*self*
into the fire instead, how to
enlist the assistance of dwarves
and princes for rescue. Before,
death was a fairy tale that would
never actually happen to us.
What liars our parents were!
The bogeyman is *too* real!

That's not just the pounding of our hearts
when we discover another questionable
mole. It's him on horseback,
his hoof beats aiming our way
to scare right into us, living hell.
We stick out our tongues, bare claws,
make like gargoyles, trying to protect

this sanctuary of our blood and breath
and drive off the monster another little while.

DRILL

Sometimes it's better for your teacher to be mean so you
don't attach to him.
   Shuryu Suzuki

When I felt the life force quickly
draining out of me, I went to her
whose ideas I'd prized and
whose laugh, when I met her,
crackled with energy.
By reputation, she was venerable,
so – I assumed she was wise,
took for granted her understanding.
Of anyone alive, she might
help me form a catch basin
to stanch, for a time,
and trap the outflow.
She ordered: *Tell me your life story.*

She heard it only as blows –
father's suicide, family murders, addictions,
struggles (vocational, marital),
depression, cancer – and
waved away my protestations
that angels had attended me
at every juncture.
With each new chapter her brow
furrowed further.
She shook her head, frowned,

and dismissing me, said,
Too much bad luck. Too much!
I can't take you on.
I won't live long enough to help you.

Not even sorry!
I gulped until I could flee,
then broke down and wept
for a full two hours.

In a couple of days it started,
at first in titters, then it built to
full-bellied guffaws.
I looked around.
What a treasury of friends!
Wise women and kind. Good men.
I looked within – more
help than anyone could need.
Her refusal had been a drill.
It bored through that last
layer of rock to the aquifer,
the well in me finally filling,
a source of my own to draw on,
a spring shooting up and up.

JESSIE

for Jessie Greenbaum
with deep gratitude

In her room the light is low.
A summer breeze puffs out
the gauzy curtains.
She is calm, calm as the sea at dawn,
and slight.
Her eyes are deep-set and steady.
Gregorian chant is softly playing.
There is a picture of poppies
in the Japanese style
taped to the ceiling.

I undress
and lay my body
between two soft sheets,
as if it were an altar,
on her table.
Utterly exposed,
without defenses entirely,
I put into her hands myself.

She is the only one
who can, without flinching
touch the scar
and with her fingers
unclench the tension,
ease its coiled larva

into flight,
restoring in just two sessions,
full range of motion
to my right arm.

Then she addresses the fear.
It has lodged itself in my flesh
like a varmint on the run,
gone into hiding.
It gnaws on me to stay alive.
She kneads the muscles of my back
as if to chase it,
sometimes using the length of her forearm
the force of her whole tensile self.

Then she picks up my feet,
cradling my heels for many minutes,
many minutes in her palms.
She does the same with my head.
I'm shaking almost violently.
Something gives way.
The fear flees,
finding my body no longer
hospitable.

In this sanctuary she has made,
receiving her ministrations,
I can almost believe
I'll be able to trust
my ashes to the earth,
that it will hold me,

take me unto itself
and use me
for the growth of other lives.

DRUM

*For Wayne Manthey
and Lora Matz*

How could she make one
when she was so weak from the chemo
she could hardly
hold up her bald head?
They said it would do her good,
and something in her
told her she must.
Where would she find the strength
to cut and stretch the wet skin,
the skill to punch with the awl
right-sized holes in it –
she'd always been all thumbs
at things like this – to lace
the raw hide in and pull it tight,
pull it tight over the frame,
to make it resound at her touch?
It was hard. It took all day
and she was whipped.
For two days more,
she couldn't play it.
It had to dry. That was fine.
She didn't think she'd ever
have the oomph or the nerve.

But then a stick by the lake
came right to her hand.

She topped it with a pocket
of buffalo wool. Walnut dye
made patterns on the head:
tongues of flame, a spray,
a hand reaching up – any or all.
To play it meant to register
desire, to pray for her life.
Still turbaned, she began
to make a sound
that was hers, over and over
two shorts followed by one long,
to feel it reverberate in space,
to hear it resonate with that
of the ancients, "primitives"
who drummed
to drive back the dark,
to come into its rhythm,
make peace with its power.

By beating this thing made of beings
once alive: the tree, the road-killed deer,
she raised the sap up through her body's trunk.
For others too who were ill,
she struck back, struck the drum for their health.
Fear flew. She moved from pattern to pattern,
into pause, into silence and out
to show her heart had not stopped
pounding. No! It had not!

BEING MEAN

Go to bed, instead of listening to a reiterating friend's
  two more hours of monologue.
Say no to going way out of your way to do an errand
  for an able relative.
Stop calling someone who never calls herself,
  giving gifts to those who don't in return,
  giving gifts to those who put you down.
Stop choosing and buying gifts
  for others to send as their own.
Refrain from coming up with suggestions
  for someone who never takes them.
Say NO to at least *half* the requests you feel
  you should respond to.
Don't jump up when still weak and cook from scratch
  a multi-course meal for the next one ill.
Let someone else.

Certain stringent measures are required
to regain and preserve your health.
Concentrate within you every healing energy.
Stare out the window. Sit with the cat in your lap.
Don't lift a finger! Except maybe to doodle.
Sip hot, soothing tea and rest.
Guard it! It's your only life,
and no one else *can*.

HINGE

On me the door swings
open, shut.
From here,
I have a great vantage
of the inner
and outer worlds.
Here. And there.
I can see how hard it is
to leave
the cushioned familiarities,
the carpets, cups
the intimates – all known.
No one *wants* to reach
this threshold
though some step up to it
desperate, resigned.
I wish all could see
the glimpses I have
of the light, its *flood*,
the tender leaves
unfurling
off whose tips
drip green words
the wind sets to song,
strange music
in a tongue not understood
until you cross…

COMING OUT WITH IT

When you feel death's hot breath
on your neck, *bad* breath,
rank, naturally, with rot,
it can just cough your life
right up out if you. What
were you saving it for *anyway?*
A special occasion? Your funeral maybe?
Why did you keep it so long
like some haughty, hoarding divinity
swallowed down in you?
That beaded purse wrapped in tissue,
antique, every last tiny glistening bead
sewn on one at a time
with such attention to detail:
four different greens to catch sunlight
shadowed over the leaves of the rose:
stashed in this recess
lined with turquoise patterned silk,
are rolls and rolls of cash
you never knew you had. That's right,
wads of large denomination bills.
They're hot. You've got to unload them –
fast! Make your deposit into the hands
of anyone passing you
or you'll get nabbed, clamped
and never have the chance to feel yourself
in the flow

of rivers and seas
and rills, Spring released, racing down mountains,
of clouds and wind-tousled trees
of giving way, un-grasping, not trying to stop
your modulation into the key tuned
to music for the molecule dance,
the rhumba going on
even in stones
even in bones of those long gone.

RENOUNCE AND ENJOY

– what Gandhi said when asked to sum up his life in three words

The road ahead,
the dreamed-of trip,
the mountaintop house,
the elusive love,
absolute fitness,
the to-die-for job,
a perfect Christmas,
obsessions, possessions,
another chance,
your worst habit,
your best shot,
your ideas, your fear,
your teeth, your bones,
your nouns, your life,
renounce.

Renounce and enjoy.

Enjoy
breathing, peeing
being
without a title,
tasting sourdough,
the movements of clouds
watching a friend talk,
rain steaming off hot sidewalks,
being in stitches, stenches,

seeing red, after a bath
having red toes,
hearing your daughter smile,
scraping, scribbling,
scrubbing – sobbing,
taping a package,
rubbing your lover's belly,
verbs, yes, and dying,
giving your all.

CONVERGENCE

In the market, the organic market where
we can find healing, untainted food,
they called out my name with gusto.
I looked over. I didn't know them.
Whose were those radiant faces?
They shouted: *It's Jean! It's Ruth!*
I'd never seem them with their *hair!*
Only bald and turbaned from the chemo.
Only gaunt, quiet, braving tentative smiles.
Now pouring from the tops of their heads
fountains of gold and silver – silken, curled.
One with each arm, I embraced them both,
felt them warm against me, wet-faced,
torsos shaking with laughter.
We are still here.

ELM

No wonder the Celts worshipped trees
and based their language on them.
I am part Celt and if I have to
live in a city, which I wish I didn't,
I can't believe my luck. We didn't even
notice, when we bought the house,
that out back, across the alley, our view
is of a strapping American elm.
I thought there weren't any left,
that they'd all been infested and had
succumbed to a fungus insinuated
into their bark by Netherlandic beetles.
Twice three stories in height, this survivor,
triumphant, of blight or its dodger,
towers over us, rises out of the ground,
a fountain, a fan, a huge sheltering umbrella.
So like a font, it's easy to see how it could be
taken for the source everything springs from
or at least the source's symbol, how anything
said might have to form in its roots
and pass through the channel of its trunk.
It could be the quintessential picture of utterance,
of words gushing out of earth's mouth.
Many-elbowed, it outdoes itself branching out
like a Hindu goddess or any good hostess
offering what she's got. Here. Some shade
to cool you. Have green, have comeliness.

How about intricacy, gravitas? Can you resist
royal comportment combined with party down?
In May it looks like a vase displaying
a long-stemmed bouquet or a reveler sporting
a ceremonial headdress, but it may be
most resplendent when bare, a lacery, manifold.
No one of our window frames can contain it.
My guardian, my *axis mundi*, it teaches:
Ignore rumors of your own extinction.
Beat the odds! Or at least play them.
Just when you think you've reached your limit,
spill over it. You're not dead yet, so stay rooted,
take nourishment, keep reaching into the blue.

TROUBLE

I've never had to look for trouble.
It's always had my number and called –
often, very devoted this kid –
and at the most inconvenient moments:
just before I'm having guests,
at 4 AM, while I'm making love.
Or it barges right in without knocking
and wipes its grimy feet on my new rug.
It's always known right where I am
and how to get to me, so when I hear
friends in mid-life talk about the need
"to create challenges for themselves,"
how they jump out of planes, climb
Kilamanjaro, run marathons, change
jobs, enter *another* doctoral program
or adopt a late-in-life child, I just
sigh and smile. I don't have to worry.
I save all the effort they put out,
remembering that the word "trouble"
comes from the word for "crowd,"
disorderly crowd. Not to worry,
another form of it will come along:
there's always a backup. I know Death will
nose around again among those I love –
Death and Trouble are bosom-buddy cousins –
or someone I was afraid might, will do me wrong.
I'll lose a limb, a gig or have way more

work than I can handle, all of it due in
RIGHT NOW, and I'll get so tired
I can't budge. More dry rot will be found;
The bottom will drop out
or I'll drop down to it – another bad biop –
or something else I've never even thought of.
Trouble is wily.
It's good at choosing the corner
you don't look in, the one you've forgotten.
I have every confidence in it.
It's the ONE thing I can count on!
I've come to expect it, stopped trying
to fend it off. After all, if so many
people are chasing it, it must be pretty HOT!
No plot without conflict, no muscle
without resistance, without the torturing
grain, no pearl. Without ferment bread
would not rise, water would never
become wine. Pain's spade digs deeper
to swell the capacity of the well,
so the seedling has a chance at growth.
It keeps us from being shallow.
Trouble then, might be the handmaiden
of miracle. So I take comfort.
I don't have to seek it out.
When it arrives, I invite it in
and ask it to sit down.
I ask what it has for me this time.
It hands me a new jam, a jar of hand-picked
blackberry which proceeds to explode
all over my clean white blouse. What

was I thinking? I should have worn old clothes,
worn goggles to protect my eyes from flying glass.
It must be rusty on proper canning procedures.
I suppose I can pick out the shards,
carefully, apply band aids, throw out the blouse.
Apparently, even what you've come to see
as sweet, can backfire on your bones.

INVITATION

for Polly Bunker

Come join us – Polly and Sam –
when we jump rope for joy,
or, as the case may be, shuffle or stumble,
as far down the road as we can.
We've *survived* (and we'll prove it!).
We're not shy.
We've come through *for now*
(The idea of forever's sure been smashed!)
thriving,
and much more pleased than punch.
There'll be some of that with cookies
when we're done.
There'll be balloons and bubbles
and ropes, of course, gaily colored
if you don't bring your own.
Meet us at Sam's porch Monday at 1.
Feel the sun on your skin,
your breath, your heart pumping.
Shout something at the top of your lungs!
And jump with us for those still struggling –
Margaret, Renee, Bea, Carolyn,
for those who are gone: Esther, Elizabeth,
for *anyone* hobbled by this damnable plague
that you love.
Yes, skip. By all means, *jump!*

DEATH

Aårlands Fjord
Norway, May 2001

Let it be like falling,
like slipping
deliberately
over the lip
of one of these
cloud-kissed mountain
cliffs rising
high and steep
out of the Flåm Valley;
like coming to the edge
and tumbling heedlessly
down over it; like
plunging,
plunging through
new leafing
hugging the mountainside
as pale, downy green fur;
let it be like thawing
into water
like dropping down
straight down
thousands of meters
an absolute vertical
free of every
restraint, then,
gathering strength

to launch down
further,
to surge,
to pulsate in space
generating gossamer
spray,
pounding, beating
until, sometimes,
with the sheer force
of downfall,
the rock beneath
will cleave;
then,
let it go
slower,
sliding over boulders,
shining them
with liquid,
sheets and showers
shooting at varying
speeds, never-ceasing
movement
white
as the first star's heart,
as the heart in torture
turning – no worries
anymore about pain.
Water cannot break.
May it be like letting
the long hair of your life
down completely,

shaking it, rippling it
like the rope Rapunzel
grew to make her
escape, and, at the bottom,
falling, at last, like
the long lost,
into the froth, into
the fjord's
emerald embrace
and charging as
thundering steeds
to the sea.

THE BENEFITS OF DISMEMBERMENT

"Myths of violent dismemberment are often referring to a
psychological good, to creation of a world of consciousness."
George R. Elder

The demon goddess has been slain,
her vast, voluptuous body,
her insufferable love chopped into lots,
her curves disbursed or cordoned off.
The fathers are greatly relieved.
Each chief has a trophy chunk,
a piece of real estate, proof of his power
and consciousness of it, over beauty,
over tenderness, vivacity, fertility unbridled.
Yes, a thigh to the overseer of the field –
he'll use it as a stool. A breast each
to the chairmen atop their obelisks.
They've had them bronzed, encased
in transparent rectangles.
From India, Babylon to Mexico, Connecticut,
their fears of usurpation have been allayed.
With Putana, Tiamat, Coyalxauhqui,
wood-chipped Helly out of the way,
their heads have cleared.
They can once again think straight –
nothing wavy, no irregularities.
Such thinking, however, is actually beclouding
and does not allow the patriarchs to hear
mouths opening at the cuts, mumbling
to one another their pain, in a language

weapon-wielders consider trivial,
rumbling, erupting in a tower-toppling
wake-up quake. The wizards have forgotten
what their own research uncovered:
each cell contains full knowledge
of all the others, contains within it
an image of the whole. Heads up!
She is rearranging herself,
reassembling for greater strength.

OBLATION

after a Yoruba sculpture

She holds her breasts in her hands;
kneeling, she offers them up.
For what better can she give the gods?
Her womanly ripeness pointed and lush
the abundance of the mother
to evoke divine fervor and favor.

One of my hands is empty.
In the left is nurturance, comfort:
a blueberry pie, sympathy, succor.
When I cannot give, I become
uneasy. I start to squirm.
I must have something to bring,
something of substance
or I don't know who I'd be.

A palm arced under absence,
a handful of air?
My right one too,
so used to taking the lead.
My face burns.
If I don't pull the hand away
in a fist of shame,
if I hold it open,
level with the other,
a nest among leafless,
truncated branches,

it is able to receive.

What is the difference
between that and begging?
And what if, without
the requisite fullness
to present, the source
of sustenance turns
its back to me
and leaves me empty?

I'll have only the knowledge
transmitted from mythic kin
that everything truly new
begins, has to, in a crying void.

RUBEDO

when the poppy lets go I know it is to lay bare
his thickly-seeded black coach
at the pinnacle of dying.
      Tess Gallagher, "The Red Poppy"

My teacher told me one thing,
Live in the soul.

When that was so,
I began to go naked,
and dance.
      Lal Ded (14th Cen.), translated by Coleman Barks

ON THE MARCH: A LIFE

Her child's heart marched with them
on TV to Montgomery from Selma,
then her young self, having caught
the drift of Watts smoke,
marched into Harlem
for fair housing and kicking heroin.
For ten candlelit, black-armbanded
miles through towns around her
college, she marched NO
to Kent State, to Cambodia's invasion.
On the White House sidewalk,
against our part in Vietnam
she marched, singing "Kum By Ya,"
off to jail, off to fasting.
To protest her school's apartheid
investments, she marched
right out of graduation.
Up bestreamered streets
she marched with vets,
then, at the gazebo, gave the prayer
to honor a small town's fallen.
A little daughter on each hand,
alongside Nagasaki citizens
against the Bomb
she marched with another million
through Manhattan's canyons;
with two of her students, rape victims,

through the campus, into the night
to safen it for all women.
For pro-choice with her teenage daughter,
her daughter's friend, she marched
down the Mall's length in Washington.
Through blossoming laurels,
rallying Earth Day 25, she hiked
to prevent developers from taking bites
out of her state's largest park.
In solidarity with friends
she marched arm-in-arm Gay Pride
down the city's widest boulevard.
Shivering mornings she marched
with placards back and forth outside
a local land mine manufacturer.
Minus one breast, with her daughter,
and masses of pink-shirted others,
she marched for a cure
from the shopping center
through suburbia.
For thirty blocks, ten below,
solstice eve, she marched
in memory of the year's
homeless, nameless dead.
From Cathedral to Capitol
she cut, with thousands
of others, a wide swathe against
war in Iraq. Because early on
her family shattered; because
for them the Dream failed;
because she lost her home

and, for awhile, her health,
she joined and joins with others,
broken and broken open
trooping through the streets together,
a force for kinder courses
history could take and hold.

PHANTOM

As with any other amputated limb
the lost breast sometimes feels "there,"
jouncing alongside its twin
as I take a stab again
at a daily constitutional.
Or it will appear in reveries
receiving attentions from
an equally phantom lover.
How the psyche compensates,
keeps groping to be whole!

Why do I dream every few months
of finding that my long-dead mother
has been living all this time
in an obscure suburb?
Laying my cheek in gladness
against her breast,
I wake only to my pillow.

Less than a week after the attacks
sculptors devised columns of light
to replace the fallen towers.
Nothing can make up for such devastation,
but we are compelled to be fooled.

From now on I will imagine rising
from the ground zero of my chest cavity

an illuminated mound. When it gets dark
and the *Race for the Cure* is over
for this year, I will see glowing
under the pink tees of other survivors
luminarias borne quavering
into a stricken, hope-hungry world.

FOODS OF A LIFETIME

That "mile high" welcome-to-town lemon meringue pie
Sweet corn, beefsteaks, Blue Lakes, minutes from the field
Those dark chocolate communion wafers, Droste's pastilles
Chopped cilantro, sour cream over Brazilian beans and rice
Jujubees, Giant Sticks, licorice at Grand Avenue Cinema
After all night childbirth: cornflakes, coffee, toast
After the flu, just a buttered baked potato
Olives, dolmades under a taverna's bougainvillea
Chutney from cranberries scrounged this afternoon
Buckle, boureg, arugula, rumaki, sauteed morelles
Goulash, paprikash, pasta, Sundays' mapled waffle wells
Still warm home fried donuts, sugared, with cinnamon
Steak, au gratins, garden chard with onions, ice cream,
your uncle's hand cranked July 4th peach – farewell meal.

VISIT

I feel like I just got here, and now I have to go.
When you're only a short while in a place,
a beautiful place you've never been
and won't see again, an island near mountains,
time goes fast. You can watch it.
Those days stretching out before you in the beginning,
spacious and pregnant, filling with plans, dwindle
                                              quickly to one.
The forsythia that sang yellow on your arrival,
as the breast of an unfamiliar western version
of a bird you know, is already greening.
Just as you bring him, perched on the topmost
branch of a fir, into focus,
                            he has flown.
You can watch the sun twinkling on the water
slip behind shifting clouds and splash the sky
tanager red before it's down.
                            Where did it go?
And the moon, plumper, no longer crescent
and cradling dark possibility, is that much closer
                                              to waning.
Of all the books you brought, you've had time
to dip into only two. When you look up from one,
the log you just put on is ash.
Time is a fire ever-moving to consume.
And the back shore you never got to explore...
Every minute is a grain of sand, a sweet, infinitesimal,
abrasion passing through you as you pass through.

TOAST

It's worth getting up for.
Just at dawn, on a dead-of-winter walk,
I could smell it wafting from homes
all around the lake as they
emerged from the dark like loaves
from an oven, steaming.
Is there an aroma more divine
than that of bread warming, bread
browning, crisping for the spread
of butter and marmalade, the sprinkling
of sugared cinnamon? Whatever
terrors the night might harbor,
how bad can it get, if hot slices
stack our morning plate, the white
ones patterned with cobalt blue?
It's what in the current vernacular
we'll all eventually be: a pleasant
redolence rising and haloing
a roughed up, frozen expanse –
for such days, we make
not-too-burnt offerings of thanks;
we raise our glasses of juice.

AGATE HUNTING

Guemes Island
for Julie Neraas

I don't really know what I'm looking for.
How do you tell them from other rocks?
I can't find a book on agates
and no one here seems sure
about how to describe them.
They say they're clear and sometimes
oddly shaped. You can almost
see right through. Local lore says they're
crystallized air pockets, the dictionary
striped or clouded quartz. I'm confused.
One native reports she can go for weeks
of walking the shore without seeing one,
then suddenly – a whole cache.
Her kids collected tons in jars.
I walk and walk looking not
at the snowed Cascades, the other
San Juans, the undulating Sound,
but down. All stones shine when wet
but when you get them home
they're dry and duller, their surfaces matte.
Though each attracts in some way
by shape or marks or color.
I keep at it. Isn't that our nature?
To keep searching for gem-like things
that stand out from those around them?
I'm afraid before I leave this island

I won't find one. When will I ever
come back? It's awful in a whole life
never to find what you want.
But, on this last day, I catch on
and reach for a carmel-colored stone,
following a tip on tone I first ignored.
I pick it up and hold it to the sun
finally out from behind almost
continuous clouds. Eureka! a word
invented for just such an moment,
for coming upon gold.
Through it I see my finger's shadow,
within it patterns and lines, nebulae, novas.
There's satisfaction in finding what we sought.
No wonder agates are objects of a hunt!
I'd only hope from all my seeking to become
as solid, not blocking but allowing light
to illumine the mystery contained within me
and pass right through.

SUSTENANCE

The branches are splitting their sides,
tiny spears of new green poking out,
and an overnight rain has sprouted
droplets along them, translucent fruit,
sparkling berries I would pluck
before the sun greedily
consumes them all himself.
This is what I live on.
This and the sound last night of peepers,
a million maracas, rattling the earth – fiesta wild,
Once more, shocking pink swatches of cherry,
red-as-the-first-time tulip grails,
a swathe of cloud pulling reluctantly
as a lover away from the side
of an island mountain, and you,
your voice over miles saying, Right now,
I'm imagining myself inside you.

DARLING

I'm still too shy to call you that
anywhere but in a poem.
Darling, the party is raving on;
the century's just about over.
It's the longest night of the year,
and it feels like it here in the
corner I'm wedged into shouting
over the combo's rendition of
"Can't Help Lovin' that Man of Mine"
the locations and occupations of our daughters
to someone I've never met and will
never see again who is already forgetting
what I'm telling him, casting an eye
around the room for another willing-enough
subject to regale with the plans for his
"little" Mies vander Rohe-like "cottage,"
lots of glass, on 6000 feet of shoreline,
deep anchorage. How wonderful for you,
I said to him, just before he stopped
his 20 minute monologue to ask, out of
politeness, about our children.
And I meant it, if it gives him happiness.
Though could it or anything be more wonderful
than even the thought that when all this
noise and fuss dies down, which, after all,
our hosts are only throwing up against
the cold out of gladness that despite the ravages:

divorce, disease, disaster, we're still here
sporting our red cummerbunds and sequined
jackets, coming as close as we can
at this point to "boogie" – could any of it
be more wonderful than knowing
that after almost 30 years I still get to
go home to our deeply mortgaged house
with you, the handsomest man here,
that we'll undress our much less than perfect
bodies and come together between flannel
sheets, if not so quickly and easily as once
we were able, yet with a starburst of love
that wins from the darkest dark all the glory
it can render? This, in the midst, with you
across the room in a clutch of acquaintances
and strangers, is what I wanted you to hear.

SEX WITH ONE-BREASTED WOMAN

He says it makes no difference
but never touches the scar, swerves
to avoid it like a right-in-the-middle-of-the-road
pothole. And she can't quite bring herself
to ask him. How can she?
She has trouble loving it herself.
Her eyes veer from it when
she looks in the mirror, as they did
this morning at the store out of shame
and deference from the tucked-up
sleeve of a landmine victim.
Instead he gives the one remaining
furious attention, sucking it
to a soreness she cherishes, grateful
for the arousal got no how else.
What if she should also lose this other?
"It" has been no impediment to full-blown
love, does not affect his potency.
In spite of this grave imperfection
she still comes and comes and comes.
But what if like Beauty, they grew,
through patient acquaintance, out of their fear?
What if they could meet this ugliness and be moved
by its pathos, could embrace it and
draw it wholly into their deepest intimacy?
What spells might break? What dimension
open out from the repulsion to make room
for a union, as yet unimagined, far greater?

WATCHING THE RIVER

There is no river like this one,
the one you visit again and again
when you're passing through.
It bubbled up out of a field
at the beginning without reason
and flows right through the town
where you entered the world and grew.

I have almost always lived near rivers:
Wabash, Missouri, Mississippi,
Hudson, Housatonic, Saugatuck, Susquehanna.
When I moved away to the place without rivers,
the worst happened.
Everything was smashed,
so I moved back
to water moving over mud.
It stitched me together
with its liquid thread.

It is the color of earth
and carries the earth with it.
It nurtures and cleanses
the body of the land,
the body of the nation
like sap through branches,
like branches of blood. Forbid it
that the river should be trashed.

It can rise
and it has
to cover our town
and bring all we've made to ruin.
It cradles our history on its bottom:
the town founder's printing press
promoting free soil and slavery's end
hurled into it by angry, landowning rebels
among the pots and arrow tips of natives
whose practice was to sit together
every day on its banks and watch the river,
watch it move.

It is always moving, moving fast.
It is always moving
like time. It never stops.
Patterns etch themselves,
as we do, on the surface of the water.
Mandalas erupt; their circles break,
break into crescents.
The crescents break up.
Briefly there is an arc of wings.
It cannot hold. Nothing does.
It never does.

Strands wind into skeins,
separate, veer away.
Dissolve.
New patterns emerge, always
new ones, similar but not like
any before: dimples, rippling,

pleats, creases, furrows.
The river is rumpled clothing
being taken off.

When I stand on these banks,
the current surges through my blood.
I feel the tributaries of my parents,
their dashed aspirations,
and their parents, their parents' parents,
wanting to establish themselves,
feeding into me, joining with my husband,
that distant, foreign system of his own
dividing into my dreams, my children
passing through me down beyond.

I will take off the clothes of illusion,
the illusion of success, of triumph.
Instead, I will watch the river.
I will see how alive it is with death
and sit down here among the cottonwoods,
their seed puffs drifting like regenerative smoke,
and do nothing but watch it go.
It will be my only profession.
Downstream from the culture,
adrift from its traditions,
how long, will I last?
Will I be alone?

MEMORIAL

Even before they've left the sanctuary
and snaked into the parish hall lured by
the thought of the chocolate cake they glimpsed
as they entered through the vestibule,
the smell of fresh coffee and casseroles,
they've forgotten you. There was a moment
during the service when they recalled,
not necessarily the things you'd *hoped*,
but how you touched them, an endearing mannerism,
the bright colors you wore – and there were tears.
Your faults, unless egregious, fade
or death pans the dross of them away
leaving just the humorous nuggets.
They had to borrow tissues from each other.

But as soon as the last hymn began to swell,
they were onto the dentist's appointment
later that day, plans to repaper the bedroom,
lists wheeling and wheeling in their minds
for groceries and errands, phone calls,
and, unaccountably, how they might in new ways
caress parts of their partner's bodies that evening.

Over the food they're chatting – not about you –
but about some candidate's peccadilloes, the weather –
a warm, cloudless summer afternoon: would there be
the predicted thunderstorm later? – about why

the out-of-town minister needed a cane, about his
resonant voice, his peculiar accent, the mole
just left of his nose. Even the grandchildren,
red-faced and sobbing earlier, are laughing,
teasing and jostling their cousins.

For now they've gone back into the sheepfold,
where they huddle together to forget
that they'll ever have to join you
wherever it is you are.
They talk a little louder, talk, though unaccustomed,
with their hands, spill more of themselves,
become uncharacteristically affectionate,
just to prove they're alive.

You should have known, living in this town
as long as you did, the river of the living,
like the one three blocks down from this church
never stops for anyone. Your appearance
makes a particular impression on the water's surface,
one that resembles the indentations of a flesh wound,
the lines taken by a stem, that moments later is erased
forever as the river flows on its inexplicable course.
Inexorable movement – time, time itself – life going on.
Remember how glad you were for it all before?

THE ONLY GOLD

This black water
soon again ice
by nightfall
is not so fouled
with street grime
or choked with rubbish
the melting,
incremental,
has revealed –
gumfoil, soiled
Burger King wraps,
chits, butts, and
disposables: lighters,
razors, motor oil bottles –
it can't reflect
the sky at dusk
striking gold.
Puddles cup
day's end light like
dream coins
we dying prize
to wish for more time
or for time to expand
as, when wet,
do crumpled,
straw-paper dragons.

LEGACY QUILT

for my daughters, Emily and Enid

It's a crazy one.
Not what I would have planned.
I'd have wanted it, or thought it ought to be
neat and ordered, balanced – serene,
the stability I never had,
to keep you centered, to keep you from harm.
But in my days, no shape has ever
held for long.
My life has been shatterings, the whole of it,
blasting me off courses I set.   I can't get
the materials assembled before the wind picks up
and blows them   all to hell and gone.
The design I had in mind, one big, rose window-like
medallion,
has had to be scotched as insufficient
truth, though there is
a miniature wistful replica in one corner, and
the whole piece   strewn
with circlets of what I could do for your nurture:
pot lids from soups and stews,
rhubarb and blueberry flutes.   I can gather
odds and ends
from each attempt: snippets that
didn't get lost in the moves, postcard flashes,
fabric transfers
scattered throughout of places I took to
or that took me in as I zoomed through, scraps

of clothes,

vocations, modes I grew out of (mostly solid cottons),

threads from a cleric's robe, rent,

shreds

of the shambles

left by my parents,

the toxic hot pink taffeta remnants

of addiction and illness,

ruby silk flashes of passion, torn

organza nights,

deep purple velvet doldrums,

depressions in drill,

splashed with cheery calico, slashed

with satin strips of electric blue – folly, rick-rack, madness,

a jagged, uneasy mélange,

a harlequin hodgepodge

sewn loosely together on the run from death,

that black cambric animal

preying on all quarters.

Over it I embroider long-faded flowers from my gardens

whip in scads of tear-soaked hankies or

try to head It off with knots and coils.

Up against it I fling a web for friendships

never torn – no matter

the force of wind,

for tradition,

which I spun with effort, not

coming by it through the blood,

the spider

dropping down over the border from denim

into chintz

that you may be supplied,
                    as she is, with the weal and wile
                    to make the wages that escaped me,
            or, if they are absent, confidence in spirit,
hedging your bits with giving, with
                    arrowhead, stem, sheaf,
                            star, blanket and cross stitches
        with chains: feathered, daisy and fly,
never forgetting, here and there, fancy
                            straight stitch embellishers
            and to lace your chaos with laughter.
            The only things complete here are
                    Numerals and Alphabet
        on Shantung banners. Make of them
    what you must, can, may   and   notice
the absolute prominence of
                    yours and your father's names
            waving amid the mess, glad pennants,
    linen, gingham, percale, and the   dog
wagging her tail,
                    fluffy white, on a swatch
        of my Grandmother's lavender Scottish wool.
    In the end, with still unfinished edges – I'll never
                meet the deadline, never   fully   catch   up – all
that was accomplished was being dashed,
            was love
                    tentatively threading together
the whole mismatched clash, from which emerges
        for you and you only
                    a plain flannel heart, pale blue.

AUTUMN QUESTIONS

Why does it seem so easy for the trees
to let the wind tear loose their leaves
and disperse a whole year's effort in an afternoon?

How can leaves let themselves be
waved madly like pennants
cheering a team that can only lose?

Are their burning colors raised in protest
or celebration? Do none of them say,
Hold on! I'm not ready now to leave what has been?

Yet who can determine in such a paroxysm
in what ways pain
sharpens the experience of pleasure?

Could there be in every catastrophe
the same shivering exuberance,
a tickertape gladness at downfall?

Does heartwood know, or not at all, that death,
that necessary rest, is only for a season, the naked tree
relieved of accomplishment in the cold?

CIDER

for the Watsons: Hal, Maggie, Maura, Garth and Seth

If you didn't have three kids 5 and under,
you'd have had time to consult an orchard-owning friend
about how to prevent blight in these
bright red Fireside apples
plucked with a picker from your tree out back,
the one centered in the yard and spreading
that drew you to this house.
But it's too much to keep in your head:
all the timing and treatments with
laundry, meals, school schedules, church,
baths, nursing, diapers, stories – all
the cleanup tasks: wiping counters and spills.
We sit at your round wooden table,
moved to the yard's edge to catch
the last precious patch of October sun.
Leaves on trees encircling us are persimmon,
are butternut squash orange, Tuscan gold.

My girls just launched, one in the Big Apple,
one Down Under, I hold your littlest
face out, as he likes it, in my lap.
I squeeze him gently against my
dummy breast, the real one having been
cut from me days before he was born.
Your two others help gather apples
for the press, a magnificent contraption,
one side of your family handed down.

The skins, though candy red as the first one ever,
are stippled with black, rotted some, bruised.
Hal cuts them up, but cannot
remove all evidence of disease.
With a hand crank, everyone taking turns,
they are ground into mash. We talk
of a child suddenly, inexplicably dead,
of your unborn niece whose blood is
poisoned by her mother's transfused *in utero*.

With sweat, the screw, resembling torture
instruments I couldn't bear to keep my eyes on
at the museum in San Gimiano,
is tightened and tightened.
Nectar, pressed from the pale green flesh
flows down the chute into the catching bowl.
We pour it into glasses all around.
The liquid, undiminished by imperfections
in the fruit, is dense and exquisite,
almost unbearably sweet as gathering
in the waning light of a waxing season.
As the kids sing and jump,
"Apple cider, apple cider,
bound to make your belly wider."
down goes the color
of cinnamon, mahogany, sorrel.

THE SAME BOAT
Omnes vulnerabilis sunt...

That was the summer on the island we all fell or fell ill.
Three – a six-year-old, a young mother,
a woodworker in his prime – tumbled off their bikes
downhill. Concussions, ghastly scabs, lost teeth.
A captain, mangling his hand in a cleat, carried
his right index finger on ice to the hospital.
The queen of *joie de vivre* blackened her face
by one misstep backwards over a porch rail.
Jailed again half-dead, drunk, was the handsomest
native son. Top of her class, the Princeton pick, thin
as a reed, could not bring herself to eat.
Our friend with MS had to drop driving from her menu.
The old musician's heart almost lost its beat.
The esteemed artist started babbling
to a teddy bear in the nursing home.
The minister's blood pressure rocketed off the charts,
preventing him from presiding at the funeral
of the mellowest bon vivant in the East.
A teacher searched her once-sharp mind
in vain for the names of her children.
A bubble in the doctor's brain exploded.
A strapping lobsterman coughed blood
all over his bathroom and the financier,
the deckhand veteran found cancer
stashed in their lungs, as the heiress
lost her young husband to Hodgkin's.
In more than a few others malignancy

was detected in breasts, wombs, bowels, glands
and blood. Not a one of us was untouched.
Instinctively, we reached for each other
across normal bounds. Grudges, habits, protocols
dissolved. Our illusion developed a rent
that there must be someone among us invulnerable.
There was no one to whom we could turn.
At first the size of a cut, it deepened, with fear
to the dimensions of the wound we felt,
then hollowed and opened into the hull of a skiff
as big as the island itself. Out to sea, adrift,
no instruments to guide us, no engine, no sail, no oars,
no one on shore – was there a shore anymore? –
it became clearer as the waves rocked us
and another storm bore down, all we could do
was hold to each other, and, fumbling over the scales,
tuning to this condition, hoo and hum.

WHAT THE PHOTOS SHOWED ME

for Jila Nikpay

We cannot wholly see ourselves.
I thought I had pushed off from the bottom,
had risen, resilient, from the abyss,
but images caught on film through her lens
show, in my rounded shoulders, resignation,
my mutilated body too heavy
to haul completely up and out.
I have not bounced back.
I cannot quite smile.
But the Greek goddess drape in which
she gently suggested I wrap myself
sanctifies this half-emergent state
making it holy, almost, as redemption, escape,
folding me, like crumbling, truncated statues,
into the eternal.

SHIFT

Chips of fallen sky:
I spy them for their color,
against the lawn's new green,
the greengage green of early leaves.
Beneath the young maple,
a small eggshell cracked in half.
I assume some predator
knocked it from its nest:
raid and ravagement,
so I bring it in and set it
on the sill above my sink
as memorial – to the bird
who might have been.
Not until Fall, dreaming
above steam, scrubbing
a stubbornly encrusted casserole
following a summer
immersed in illness
does it occur that
birth is more likely
the cause of the breakage.
The bird who might now be
lifted the lid of his firmament
and, though it took
some shattering,
the old has passed away –
a new earth, a new heaven.

PASSEMENTERIE

Even those whose taste inclines
to simple lines free of ornamentation
would be hard pressed to resist
the embellishments of peak April.
The whole outdoors is a notions showroom,
an emporium of trim.

The trees are sprigged with mini-
gold-green pom-poms rah-rahing Spring,
hung with thousands of dangling tassels.
In sun, in gusts, glitzy new leaves
are dazzling spangles, sprinkling
passersby with fairy dust.

Redbud limbs are bedizened with blue-pink
piping. Pears, apples, azaleas, crabs,
cherries, lilacs, rhodies fluff up their pastel
furbelows. What a flouncing bevy!
What primping and prinking!

Greenagain lawns are fairly lame-ed.
Gold braid frames each brick of the walkway.
Only on high is such orphrey
used for paving, and drying sidewalks
are silvered with ruching, a gallooning of rain.

The elm indulges in frilly millenary
amid the frippery of constant birdsong,
over the scrolling of fancy, unfurling ferns,
the all-stops-out displays, the appliqués
of tulip, daffodil, hyacinth, iris.

It's a bit much, all this gimp and fringe,
for those with a minimalist tendency.
It's over-the-top gaudy, *très outré,*
just plain frou-frou. But for those
who have been stripped,
whose prospects are slim, prognosis
questionable, we glory in this garishment.
We're just tickled.

AS DEATH APPROACHES

I can't believe I'm laughing!
I'd have sworn I'd be
shaking or sniveling.
And I sure didn't expect
a limousine.
I've never been in a limousine.
No biggy.
I've had better than fame.
Who needs the pressure?
As for fortune, I'm filthy.
That's why I'm laughing.
I've had so much love:
the giving, the getting.
It's shameful.
It's embarrassing.
And it's too late.
No one can take it away!
And I've had the pain
to help me appreciate it.
Thank God for the pain!
Easy for me to say
now that I'm going!
But no, seriously,
the kicks in the teeth,
the gut, the rugs
pulled out, slammed doors,
setbacks, snubs.

Without them, I'd
never have recognized
Love, bedraggled,
plain eyes shining,
happy to see me.
Do I want more?
Of course I want more!
I always want more
of everything: money, hugs,
lovemaking, art, butter,
woods, flowers, the sea,
M&Ms, chips, tops, bottoms,
trips – I did give up drinking –
time, sure, and yes,
I'd like to see
my grandchildren,
if there are any.
I'd like to see my books
but more has never
been good for me anyway.
Enough – that's what I've
always needed to learn,
and is there a better way?
So this laughter
I had to work up to
through so many tears,
it just keeps coming
like a fountain, a spray.
Let it light on you
refreshment, benediction,
as I'm driven away.

BLESSING

It comes from the French, *blesser*, to wound, to spill blood,
this word that means "conducive to happiness."
No flower blooms unless it roots in mud.

If we try to get by unscathed (though no one ever does),
we'll be numb to kisses planted by the goddess.
"Blessing" from the French, *blesser*, to wound, to spill blood.

We whine and fume and shout we've had enough! –
or *never* have, priming ourselves for some dreamed efflorescence.
No flower blooms, though, unless it roots in mud.

Dust dancing in shafts of sun, sponging plates clean, the touch
of a cashier's palm, common things keen and sweeter near death.
Anglo-Saxon's *bletsian* means consecration with blood.

The gut kick, lost job/ breast/ mind, all-the-time pain, floods
plow us up and soften our ground for a Presence.
Flowers won't bloom unless they're rooted in mud.

Why fight it? Like Isaac, go humbly under divine knives, trust
they'll prune whatever checks growth. Accept the whole mess!
Gloss for *benedictus*, blessings are bliss/spilled blood, hand in glove.
Where are the roots of those brilliant red blooms? In mud!

ZOË

for Zoë Michael

Tonight I had the honor,
great honor,
of dancing with life,
a girl named Zoë, nine.
She came right up and asked me.
How could I refuse
her bright, eager eyes,
her reduce-you-to-nothing-
but-quivering-plasma smile?
Why did she choose me,
a bulky, clumsy woman
who must, to her, look old?
Because I was the only one
who appeared remotely game?
We entered the circle of clapping adults.
Stumbling at first, stepping on toes,
we mangled a waltz. She didn't mind!
Quicker than I once would have,
I decided to let her lead. Why not?
What I once thought I knew,
I've long since forgot.
We whirled through "Balalaika,"
spinning clockwise
and counter the clock.
As we went, we speeded up.
Through "Clemantine" we –
Oh my darlin' – swooped,

moving now on beat, now
off with the mandolin,
guitars, voices, bongos, piano.
Never out of breath, somehow,
but in it, buoyed and floating,
we were dancing for them all,
everyone who couldn't or wouldn't.
Her curls bounced.
Her skirt flared.
The canes, the wheelchair, the paling
of some faces around the circle,
people we both know and love,
she took them into account,
but she was not thinking of death.
It was not happening now.
She insisted we keep going
through the progressions of yet
another song as if the dance
would go on and on and on...

ABOUT THE AUTHOR

SUSAN DEBORAH KING has worked as a Presbyterian minister and psychotherapist and now teaches writing and leads retreats on creativity and spirituality. She has two previous books of poetry: *Tabernacle, Poems of an Island,* (Island Institute) and *Coven,* (Folio Bookworks), a finalist for the Minnesota Book Award. The mother of grown twin daughters, she lives with her husband in Minneapolis and on an island in Maine.

For forty years, JANE NORLING has made artwork that promotes social justice. As graphic designer, poster artist, muralist and studio painter, she combines the sensibilities of fine art with the tools of design to create imagery that strongly advocates a point of view.

After treatment for breast cancer in 1988, Jane designed publicity for the Oakland CA Women's Cancer Resource Center and has made occasional paintings on the subject of women and cancer.

"Was it Breast Cancer?" (oil crayon on canvas) emerged from a model session in which Jane imagined the model with her breast missing from cancer. The painting belongs to a close friend with metastatic breast cancer.

Jane has worked with arts, social service, electoral campaign and union organizations in the San Francisco Bay Area since 1970. She lives in Berkeley with her union activist husband Bob Lawson. Her son Rio Chavez is a musician in Chicago.

Contact Jane at www.janenorling.com.